The Ultimate Mediterranean Breakfast Cookbook

Flavorful recipes
To start the day with the right
energy

Carlo Montesanti

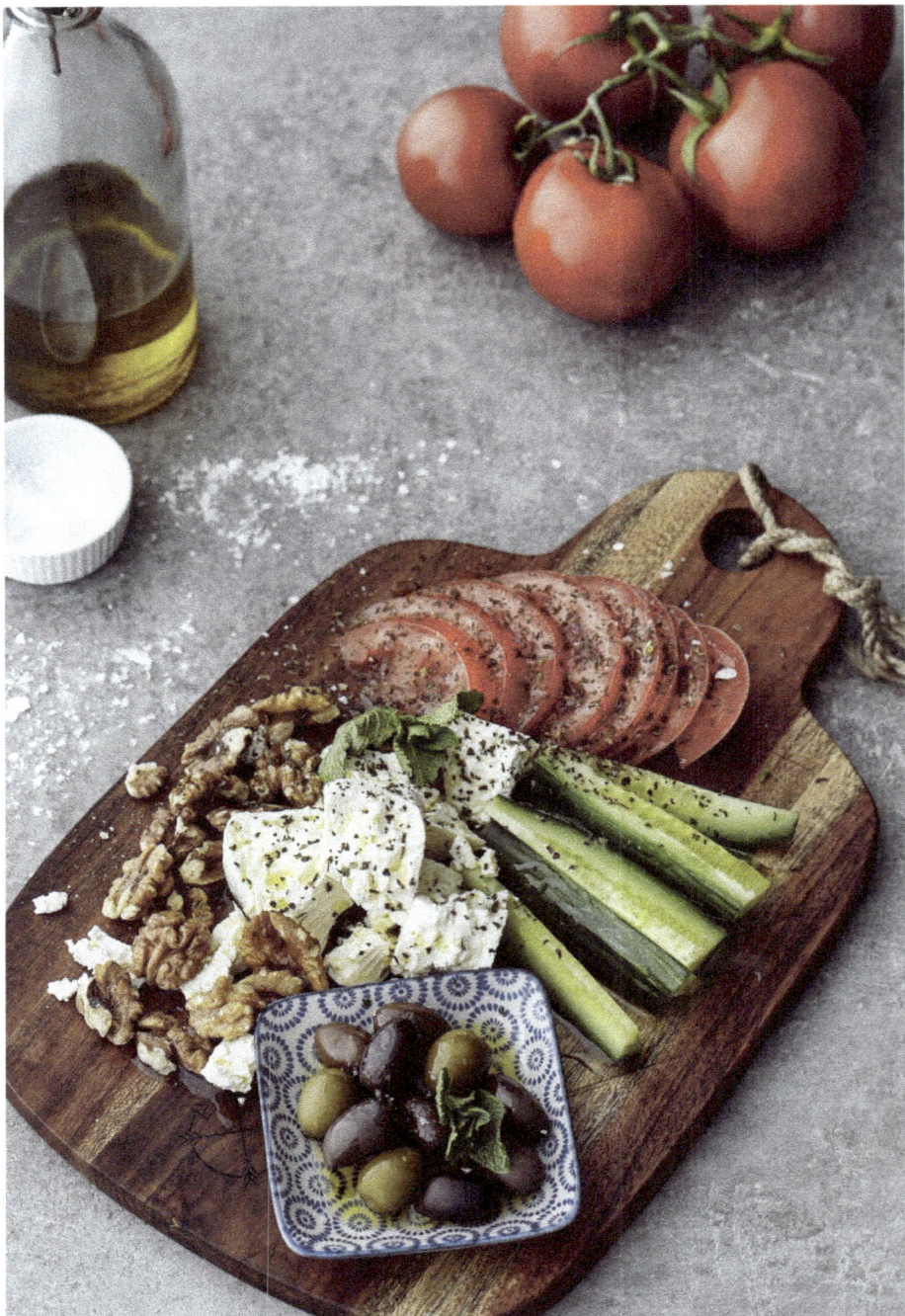

advice. the content within this book has been derived from various sources. please consult a licensed professional before attempting any techniques outlined in this book.

by reading this document, the reader agrees that under no circumstances is the author responsible for any losses, direct or indirect, which are incurred as a result of the use of information contained within this document, including, but not limited to, — errors, omissions, or inaccuracies.

Table of Contents

Multigrain Blueberry Yogurt Pancakes

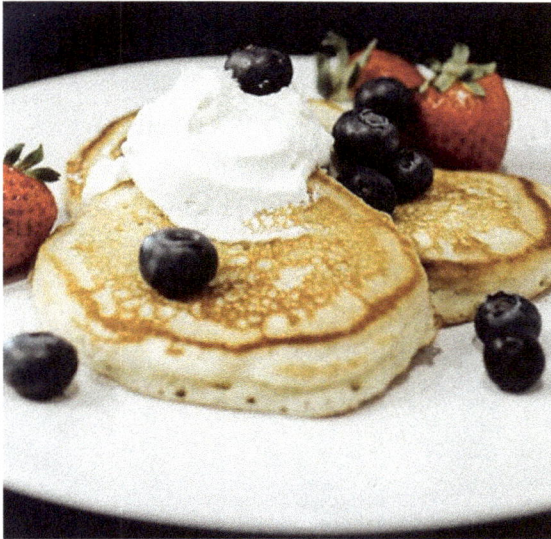

Prep Time: 10 min

Cook Time: 20 min

Serve: 12-14

Ingredients:

- Blueberries, one cup, fresh

- Eggs, two

- Salt, one-quarter teaspoon

- Plain Greek yogurt, one cup

- Baking powder, one teaspoon and one tablespoon

  Milk, four tablespoons

- Barley or rye flour, one-quarter of a cup

- All-purpose flour, one-half of a cup

- Butter, three tablespoons, melted

- Wheat flour, one-half of a cup

- Lemon zest, one teaspoon

- Vanilla, one teaspoon

Preparation:

1. Blend the milk, eggs, yogurt, and butter. Mix the dry ingredients in another bowl. Spoon the wet ingredients gently into the dry ingredients and blend. Pour the batter, one-quarter of a cup for each pancake, into the hot skillet that has been oiled with a light coating of olive oil. Cook each pancake for three to four minutes on each side.

Mediterranean Frittata

Prep Time: 5 min

Cook Time: 25 min

Serve: 6

Ingredients:

- Eggs, six

- Black pepper, one-quarter of a teaspoon

- Milk, one-quarter of a cup

- Oregano, one teaspoon

- Tomatoes, one-quarter of a cup, diced

- Salt, one teaspoon

- Green olives, one-quarter of a cup, chopped finely

- Feta cheese, one-quarter of a cup, crumble

- Black olives, one-quarter of a cup, chopped finely

Preparation:

1. Heat the oven to 400. Spray oil an eight-by-eight-inch baking dish. Beat the milk into the eggs, and then add the other ingredients. Pour this mixture into the baking dish and bake for twenty minutes.

Banana Blueberry Muffins

Prep Time: 20 min

Cooking Time: 25 min

Serve: 12

Ingredients:

- Mashed ripe banana, three-fourths of a cup

- Blueberries, one and one-half cups, fresh or frozen

- Milk, three-fourths of a cup

- Walnuts, one-half cup, chopped finely

- Apple cider vinegar, one teaspoon

- Applesauce, one-half of a cup

- Baking soda, one-half of a teaspoon

- Vanilla, one teaspoon

- Sea salt, one-half of a teaspoon

- Olive oil, one-quarter of a cup

- Cinnamon, one and one-half teaspoon, ground

- Flour, two cups

- Baking powder, two teaspoons

Preparation:

1. Heat the oven to 350. Spray oil in the twelve-cup muffin pan. Mix the vanilla, vinegar, milk, and bananas. Mix in a separate bowl the baking soda, salt, cinnamon, baking powder, and flour. Mix the wet ingredients into the dry ones. Fold in the blueberries and walnuts. Pour your batter into the muffin cups, and let it bake for twenty-five minutes.

Spiced Chickpeas Bowls

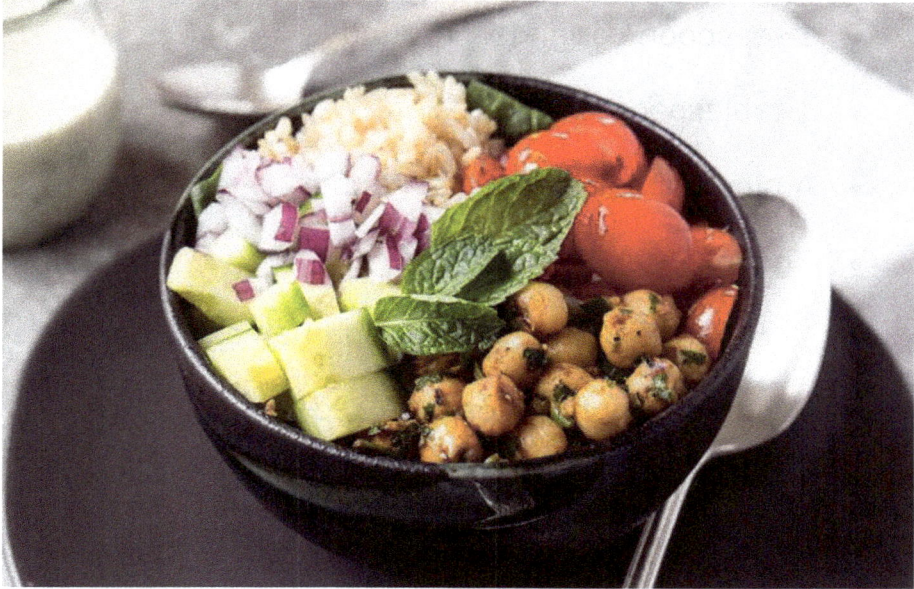

Prep Time: 10 min

Cook Time: 30 min

Serve: 4

Ingredients:

- 15 ounces canned chickpeas, drained and rinsed
- ¼ teaspoon cardamom, ground

- ½ teaspoon cinnamon powder

- 1 and ½ teaspoons turmeric powder

- 1 teaspoon coriander, ground

- 1 tablespoon olive oil

- A pinch of salt and black pepper

- ¾ cup Greek yogurt

- ½ cup green olives, pitted and halved

- ½ cup cherry tomatoes, halved

- 1 cucumber, sliced

Preparation:

1. Spread the chickpeas on a baking sheet, add the cardamom, cinnamon, turmeric, coriander, the oil, salt and pepper, toss and bake at 375 degrees F for 30 minutes.

2. In a bowl, combine the roasted chickpeas with the rest of the ingredients, toss, and serve breakfast.

Avocado Spread

Prep Time: 5 min

Cook Time: 0 min

Serve: 8

Ingredients:

- 2 avocados roughly chopped

- 1 tablespoon sun-dried tomatoes, chopped

- 2 tablespoons lemon juice

- 3 tablespoons cherry tomatoes, chopped

- ¼ cup red onion, chopped

- 1 teaspoon oregano, dried

- 2 tablespoons parsley, chopped

- 4 kalamata olives, pitted and chopped

- A pinch of salt and black pepper

Preparation:

1. Put your avocados into a bowl and mash with a fork.

2. Add the rest of the ingredients, stir to combine and serve as a morning spread.

Cheesy Yogurt

Prep Time: 4 h and 5 min

Cook Time: 0 min

Serve: 4

Ingredients:

- 1 cup Greek yogurt

- 1 tablespoon honey

- ½ cup feta cheese, crumbled

Preparation:

In a blender, combine the yogurt with the honey and the cheese and pulse well. Divide into bowls and freeze for 4 hours before serving for breakfast.

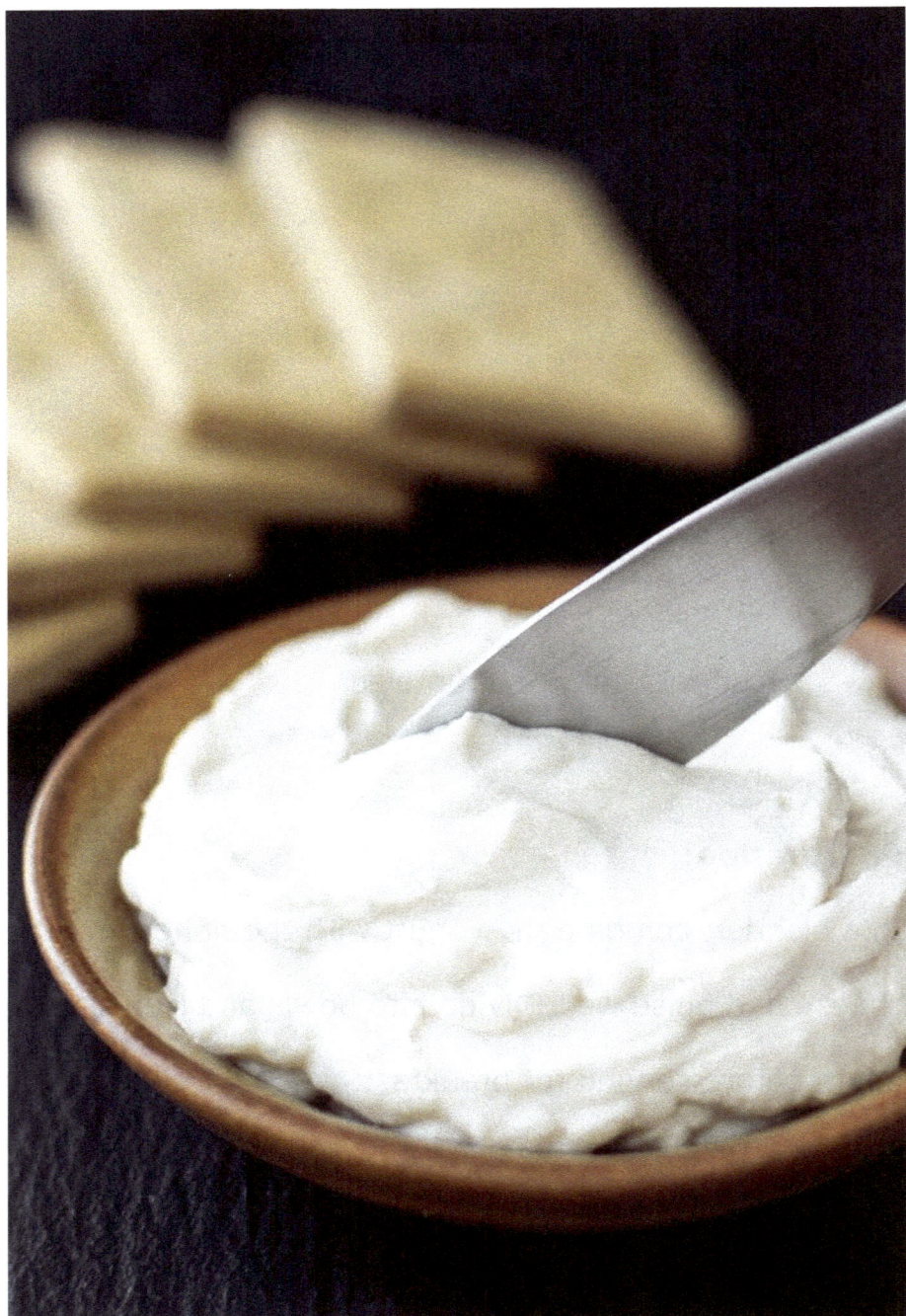

Baked Omelet Mix

Prep Time: 10 min

Cook Time: 45 min

Serve: 12

Ingredients:

- 12 eggs, whisked
- 8 ounces spinach, chopped
- 2 cups almond milk
- 12 ounces canned artichokes, chopped
- 2 garlic cloves, minced
- 5 ounces feta cheese, crumbled
- 1 tablespoon dill, chopped
- 1 teaspoon oregano, dried
- 1 teaspoon lemon pepper
- A pinch of salt
- 4 teaspoons olive oil

Preparation:

1. Heat a pan with the oil over medium-high heat, add the garlic and the spinach and sauté for 3 minutes.

2. In a baking dish, combine the eggs with the artichokes and the rest of the ingredients. Add the spinach mix and toss a bit, bake the mix at 375 degrees F for 40 minutes, divide between plates and serve for breakfast.

Veggie Bowls

Prep Time: 10 min

Cook Time: 5 min

Serve: 4

Ingredients:

- 1 tablespoon olive oil
- pound asparagus, trimmed and roughly chopped
- 3 cups kale, shredded
- 3 cups Brussels sprouts, shredded
- ½ cup hummus
- 1 avocado, peeled, pitted and sliced
- 4 eggs, soft boiled, peeled and sliced
- 2 tablespoons of lemon juice
- 1 garlic clove, minced
- 2 teaspoons Dijon mustard
- 2 tablespoons olive oil
- Salt and black pepper to the taste

Preparation:

1. Heat a pan with 2 tablespoons oil over medium-high heat, add the asparagus and sauté for 5 minutes stirring often.

2. In a bowl, combine the other 2 tablespoons oil with the lemon juice, garlic, mustard, salt and pepper and whisk well.

3. In a salad bowl, combine the asparagus with the kale, sprouts, hummus, avocado and the eggs and toss gently.

4. Add the dressing, toss and serve for breakfast.

Mediterranean Egg Cups

Prep Time: 15 min

Cooking Time: 25 min

Serve: 6

Ingredients:

- Bell pepper, one cup chopped finely

- Feta cheese, three tablespoons crumbled small

- Mushrooms, one cup chopped finely

- Eggs, ten

- Black pepper, one-quarter of a teaspoon

- Milk, two-thirds of a cup

- Salt, one-quarter of a teaspoon

- Garlic powder, one teaspoon

- Spray oil

Preparation:

1. Heat the oven to 350. Spray oil in the twelve-muffin cup pan. Add the pepper, salt, garlic powder, and milk into the beaten egg until mixed well. Add in the peppers and the mushrooms.

2. Fill the muffin pan cups with this mix. Bake for twenty-five minutes. Cool for five minutes then top with the cheese and serve.

Avocado and Apple Smoothie

Prep Time: 5 min

Cook Time: 0 min

Serve: 2

Ingredients:

- 2 cups spinach

- 1 green apple, cored and chopped

- 1 avocado, peeled, pitted and chopped

- 3 tablespoons chia seeds

- 1 teaspoon honey

- 1 banana, frozen and peeled

- 2 cups coconut water

Preparation:

In your blender, combine the spinach with the apple and the rest of the ingredients, pulse, divide into glasses and serve.

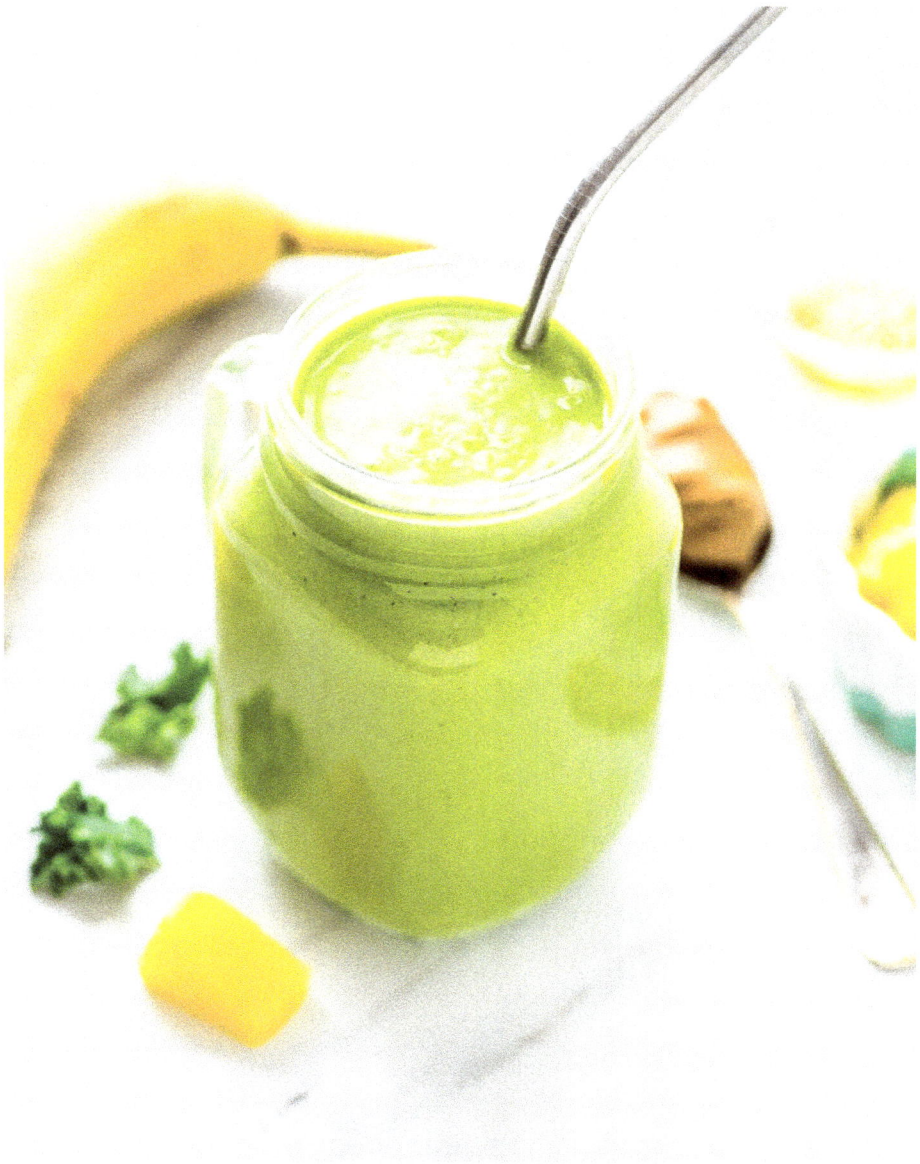

Mini Frittatas

Prep Time: 5 min

Cook Time: 15 min

Serve: 12

Ingredients:

- 1 yellow onion, chopped

- 1 cup parmesan, grated

- 1 yellow bell pepper

- 1 red bell pepper

- 1 zucchini, chopped

- Salt and black pepper to the taste

- 8 eggs, whisked

- A drizzle of olive oil

- 2 tablespoons chives, chopped

Preparation:

1. Heat a pan with the oil over medium-high heat, add the onion, the zucchini and all the ingredients (except the eggs), chives and sauté for 5 minutes stirring often.

2. Divide this mix on the bottom of a muffin pan, pour the eggs mixture on top, sprinkle salt, pepper and the chives and bake at 350 degrees F for 10 minutes.

3. Serve the mini frittatas for breakfast right away.

Berry Oats

Prep Time: 5 min

Cook Time: 0 min

Serve: 2

Ingredients:

- ½ cup rolled oats

- 1 cup almond milk

- ¼ cup chia seeds

- A pinch of cinnamon powder

- 2 teaspoons honey

- 1 cup berries, pureed

- 1 tablespoon yogurt

Preparation:

In a bowl, combine the oats with the milk and the rest of the ingredients except the yogurt, toss, divide into bowls, top with the yogurt and serve cold for breakfast.

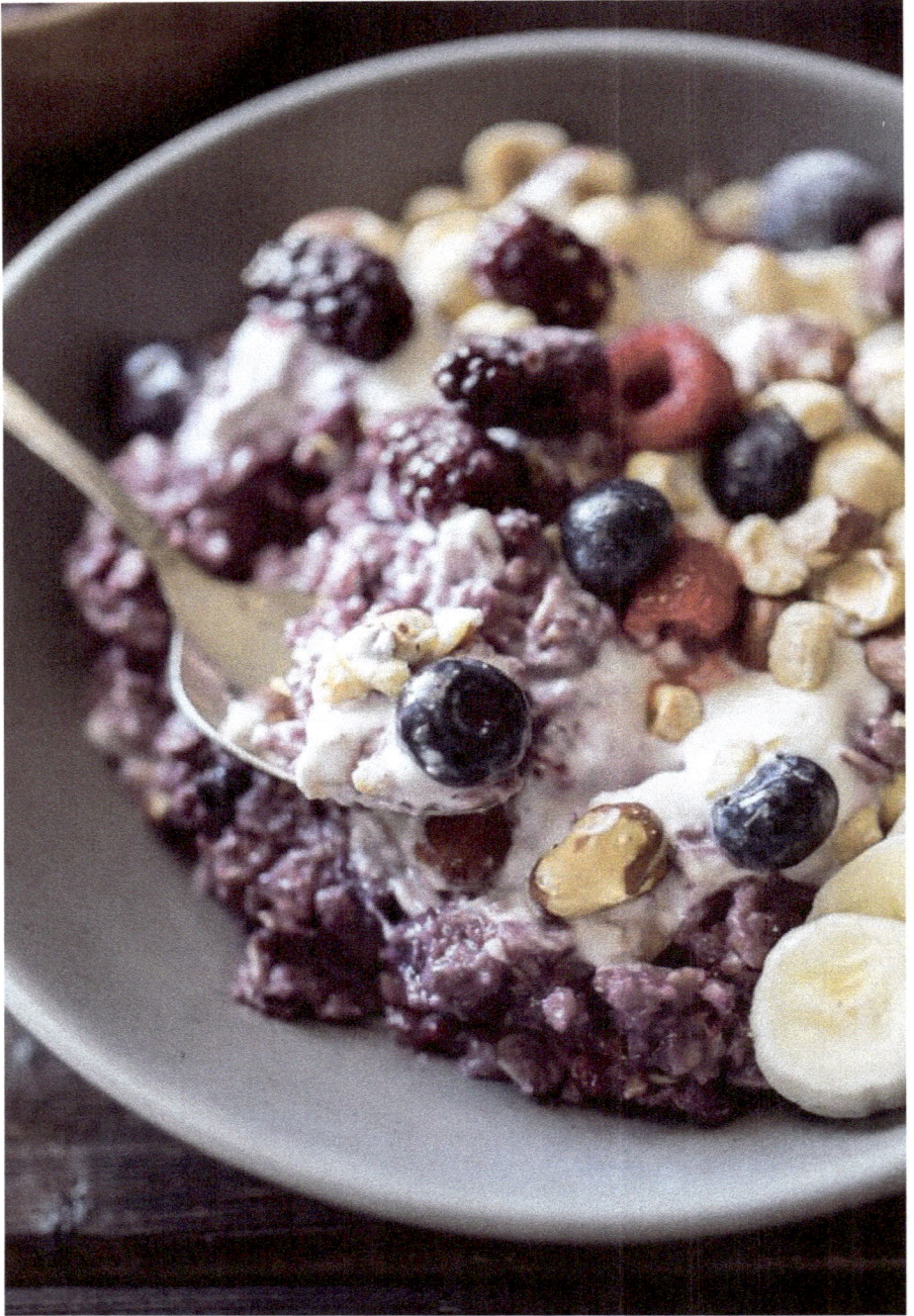

Quinoa and Eggs Pan

Prep Time: 10 min

Cook Time: 23 min

Serve: 4

Ingredients:

- 4 bacon slices, cooked and crumbled

- A drizzle of olive oil

- 1 small red onion

- 1 red bell pepper

- 1 sweet potato, grated

- 1 green bell pepper

- 2 garlic cloves, minced

- 1 cup white mushrooms, sliced

- ½ cup quinoa

- 1 cup chicken stock

- 4 eggs, fried

- Salt and black pepper to the taste

Preparation:

1. Heat a pan with the oil over medium-low heat, add the onion, garlic, bell peppers, sweet potato and the mushrooms, toss and sauté for 5 minutes.

2. Add the quinoa, toss and cook for 1 more minute. Add the stock, salt and pepper, stir and cook for 15 minutes.

3. Divide the mix between plates, top each serving with a fried egg, sprinkle some salt, pepper, crumbled bacon, and serve breakfast.

Stuffed Tomatoes

Prep Time: 10 min

Cook Time: 15 min

Serve: 4

Ingredients:

- 2 tablespoons olive oil

- 8 tomatoes, insides scooped

- ¼ cup almond milk

- 8 eggs

- ¼ cup parmesan, grated

- Salt and black pepper to the taste

- 4 tablespoons rosemary, chopped

Preparation:

1. Grease a pan with the oil and arrange the tomatoes inside.

2. Crack an egg in each tomato, divide the milk and the rest of the ingredients, introduce the pan in the oven and bake at 375 degrees F for 15 minutes. Serve for breakfast right away.

Watermelon "Pizza"

Prep Time: 10 min

Cook Time: 0 min

Serve: 4

Ingredients:

- 1 watermelon slice cut 1-inch thick and then from the center cut into 4 wedges resembling pizza slices
- 6 kalamata olives, pitted and sliced 1-ounce feta cheese, crumbled
- ½ tablespoon balsamic vinegar
- 1 teaspoon mint, chopped

Preparation:

Arrange the watermelon "pizza" on a plate, sprinkle the olives and the rest of the ingredients on each slice and serve right away for breakfast.

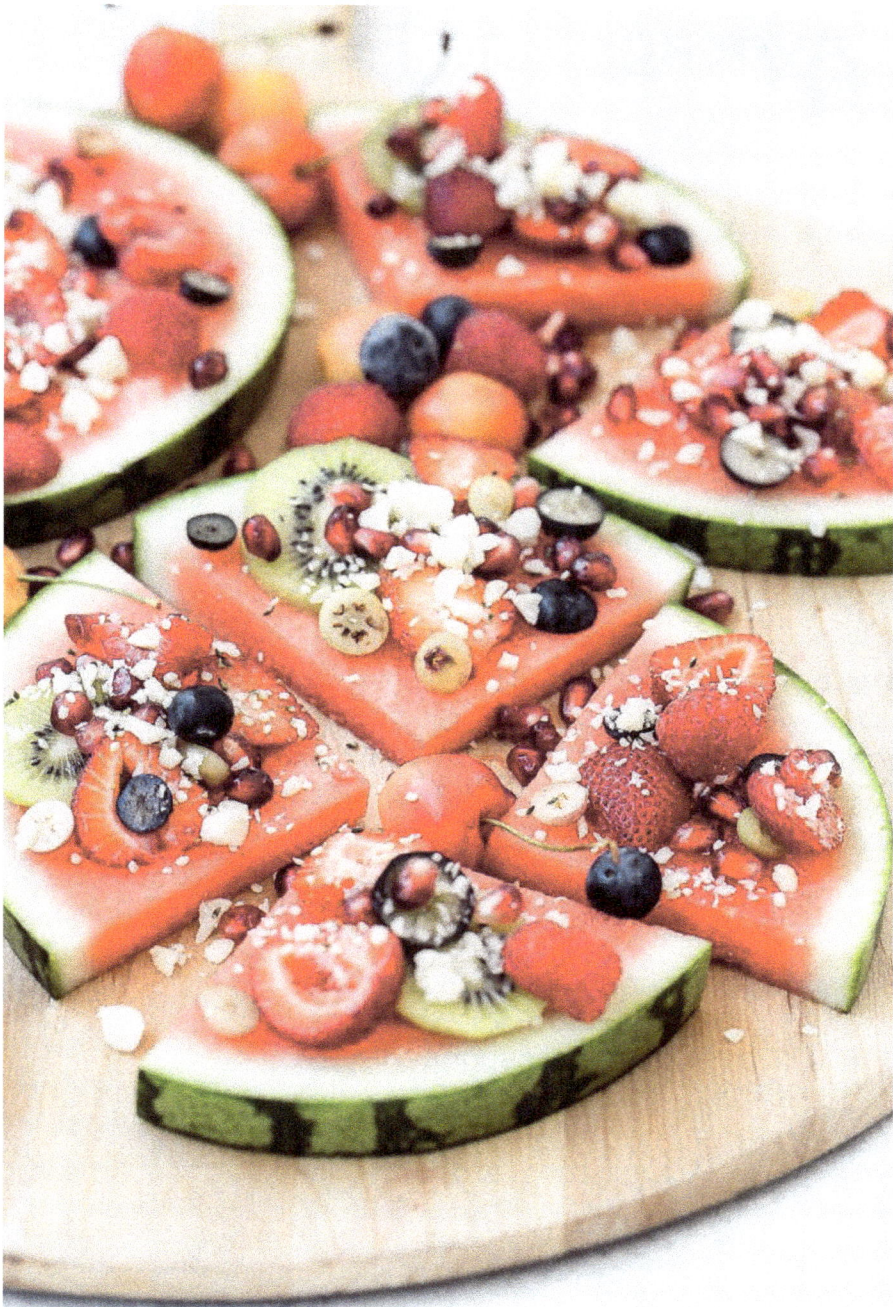

Avocado and Feta Cheese Baked Eggs

Prep Time: 25 min

Cook Time: 15 min

Serve: 2

Ingredients:

- Salt and pepper, one-quarter of a teaspoon each

- Eggs, four

- Feta cheese, three tablespoons, crumbled finely

- Avocado, one large, cut into slices

- Olive oil, two tablespoons

Preparation:

1. Heat the oven to 350. Lay the slices of avocado into two oven-safe personal- sized baking dishes. Crack two of the eggs into each bowl easily, so you do not break the yoke.

2. Add the cheese crumbles and lightly sprinkle pepper and salt in each cup. Bake them for fifteen minutes.

Greek Yogurt Pancakes

Prep Time: 15 min

Cook Time: 15 min

Serve: 6

Ingredients:

- Flour, one and one-quarter cup
- Blueberries, one-half of a cup, fresh or frozen
- Salt, one-quarter of a teaspoon
- Baking powder, two teaspoons
- Milk, one-half of a cup
- Baking soda, one teaspoon
- Butter, three tablespoons
- Plain Greek yogurt, one and one-half of a cup
- Eggs, three

Preparation:

Mix the dry ingredients and the wet ingredients separately; leave the blueberries for now. Mix wet and dry ingredients and then gently fold in the blueberries. Top the pancakes with more yogurt and blueberries if desired.

Mediterranean Eggs

Prep Time: 5 min

Cook Time: 1 h 18 min

Serve: 6

Ingredients:

- Yellow onion, one large, cut in thin slices

- Parsley, one-quarter of a cup, chopped finely

- Butter, one tablespoon

- Sea salt, one-quarter of a teaspoon

- Olive oil, one tablespoon

- Black pepper, one-half of a teaspoon

- Garlic, one clove, chopped fine

- Feta cheese, three ounces, crumbled small

- Tomatoes, one-half of a cup, cut in thin slices

- Eggs, eight

Preparation:

1. Cook the onions in the butter for about ten minutes. Stir in the olive oil, along with the tomatoes and garlic and cook for five more minutes. Lower the heat and break the eggs over the mix, drizzling with pepper, salt, and feta.

2. Cover and cook for ten minutes without stirring over low heat. Sprinkle on the parsley and serve.

Mediterranean Breakfast Salad

Prep Time: 30 min

Cook Time: 0 min

Serve: 4

Ingredients:

- Eggs, four, hard-boiled and sliced in thin slices

- Lemon juice, three tablespoons

- Arugula, ten cups, washed and dried

- Olive oil, two tablespoons

- Tomato, one large, cut into eight wedges

- Dill, one-half of a cup, chopped finely

- Cucumber, one-half of a cup, chopped finely

- Almonds, one cup, chopped finely

- Quinoa, one cup, cooked and already cooled

- Avocado, one large, sliced in thin slices

Preparation:

1. Mix the quinoa with the tomatoes, cucumber, and arugula. Add the salt, pepper, and olive oil; toss lightly.

2. Place the salad mix on four salad plates, arrange the sliced egg and the avocado slices on top of the salad mix, and top with the almonds and herbs.

3. Drizzle the lemon juice all over it.

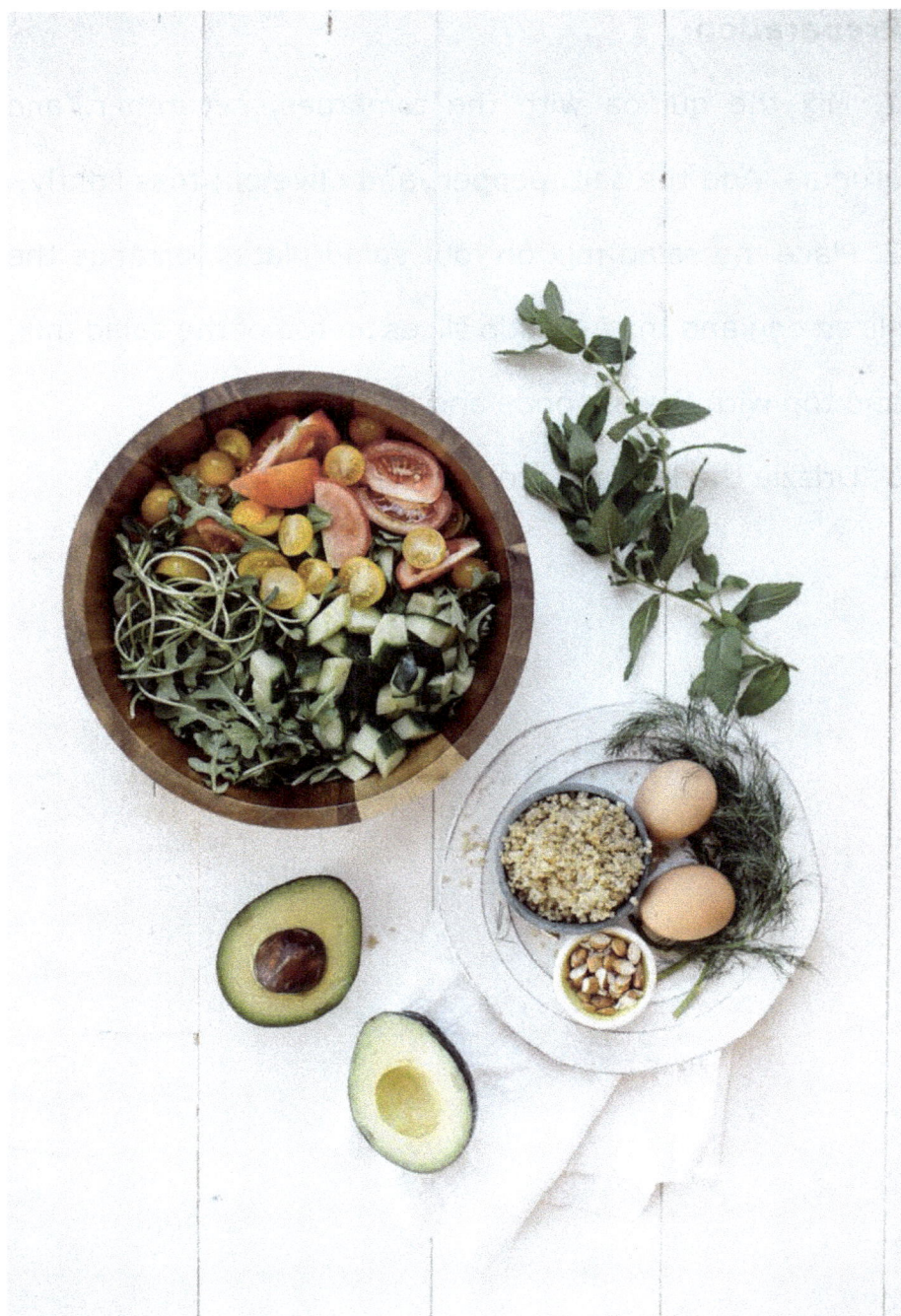

Mushroom and Spinach Omelet

Prep Time: 3 min

Cook Time: 15 min

Serve: 1-2

Ingredients:

- Olive oil, one tablespoon

- Green onion, one, diced finely

- Red onion, one-quarter of a cup, diced finely

- Egg, three

- Spinach, one and one-half fresh, chopped small

- Feta cheese, one-half of a cup, crumbled small

- Button mushrooms, five, sliced thinly

Preparation:

1. Sauté the onions, mushrooms, and spinach for three minutes in the olive oil and then set them to the side. Pour the well-beaten eggs into the skillet.

2. Cook the eggs for about 3 or 4 minutes until the edges begin to brown. Sprinkle all of the other ingredients onto half of the omelet and fold the other half over the ingredients. Cook the omelet for one minute on each side.

Southwest Tofu Scramble

Prep Time: 10 min

Cook Time: 20 min

Serve: 2

Ingredients:

- Kale, two cups, washed, dried, and chopped into small pieces

- Eggs, four, beaten well

- Red pepper, one-half of one, sliced thinly

- Olive oil, two tablespoons

- Red onion, one-fourth of one, sliced thinly

- Garlic powder, one teaspoon

- Turmeric, a quarter teaspoon

- Water, just enough to thin ingredients

- Chili powder, a quarter teaspoon

- Sea salt, one-half teaspoon

- Cumin powder, one-half teaspoon

Preparation:

1. Make the sauce, mix all of the spices in a bowl, and add just enough water to stir into a sauce-type of consistency. Cook the red pepper, kale, and onion for three to four minutes in the olive oil.

2. Then pour the beaten egg all over the mix in the pan, and cook it until the eggs reach your desired set.

Ricotta & Pear Bake

Prep Time: 10 min

Cook Time: 15 min

Serve: 4

Ingredients:

- 16 Ounce Whole Milk Ricotta Cheese

- 2 Eggs, Large

- 1 Tablespoon Sugar

- ¼ Cup Whole Wheat Flour

- 1 Teaspoon Vanilla Extract, Pure

- ¼ Teaspoon Nutmeg

- 2 Tablespoon Water

- 1 Pear, Cored & Diced

- 1 Tablespoon Honey, Raw

Preparation:

1. Heat your oven to 400, and then get out four ramekins that are six ounces each. Grease them with cooking spray.

2. Get out a bowl and beat your eggs, flour, sugar, ricotta, vanilla, and nutmeg together. Spoon this mixture into your ramekins, baking for about twenty-five minutes. The ricotta should be almost set. Remove from the oven, and let it cool.

3. While you make your ricotta get out a saucepan and place it over medium heat. Simmer your pears in water for ten minutes. They should soften, and then remove them from heat. Stir your honey in, and then serve the ricotta ramekins topped with your cooked pears.

Fruit Bulgur

Prep Time: 5 min

Cook Time: 10 min

Serve: 5

Ingredients:

- 2 Cups Milk, 2%

- 1 ½ Cups Bulgur, Uncooked

- ½ Teaspoon Cinnamon

- 2 Cups Dark Sweet cherries, Frozen

- 8 Figs, Dried & Chopped

- ½ Cup Almonds, Chopped

- ¼ Cup Mint, Fresh & Chopped

- ½ Cup Almonds, Chopped Warm 2%

- Milk to Serve

Preparation:

1. Get out a medium saucepan and combine your water, cinnamon, bulgur and milk. Stir it once and bring it just to a boil. Once it begins to boil then cover it, and then reduce your heat to medium-low. Allow it to simmer for ten minutes. The liquid should be absorbed.

2. Turn the heat off, but keep your pan on the stove. Stir in your frozen cherries. You don't need to thaw them, and then ad din your almonds and figs. Stir well before covering for a minute.

3. Stir your mint in, and then serve with warm milk drizzled over it.

Lentil Omelet

Prep Time: 5 min

Cook Time: 10 min

Serve: 2

Ingredients:

- 8 Avocado Slices for Garnish

- ½ Cup Grape Tomatoes, Chopped for Garnish

- ½ Cup Lentils, Canned, Drained & Rinsed

- 1 Cup Asparagus, Chopped

- ¼ Cup Onion, Chopped

- 1 Tablespoon Thyme

- 4 Eggs, Whisked

Preparation:

1. Get out a bowl and whisk you egg and thyme together. Place it to the side. Heat a skillet using medium heat, and cook your onion and asparagus for two to three minutes. Add in your lentils, cooking for another two minutes. It should be heated all the way through. Reduce the heat to low.

2. Get out a skillet and place it over medium heat, whisking your eggs again before adding them to the skillet. Cook for two to three minutes. They should be set on the bottom.

3. Spread your lentil and asparagus mixture on one half. Cook for another two minutes before folding the egg over the lentil filling. Cook for another two minutes.

4. Repeat with your remaining ingredients to create a second omelet. Garnish with avocado before serving.

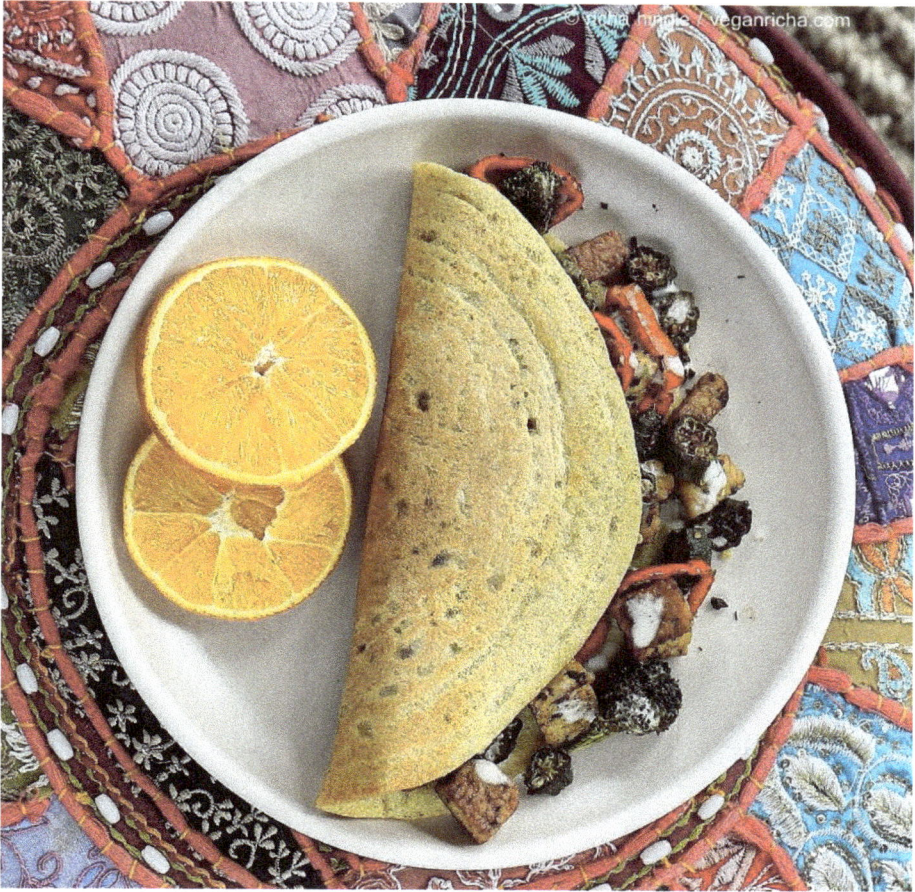

Bacon and Brussels Sprout Breakfast

Prep Time: 10 min

Cook Time: 15 min

Serve: 3

Ingredients:

- Apple cider vinegar, 1½ tbsps.

- Salt

- Minced shallots, 2

- Minced garlic cloves, 2

- Medium eggs, 3

- Sliced Brussels sprouts, 12 oz.

- Black pepper

- Chopped bacon, 2 oz.

Directions:

1. Melted butter, 1 tbsp.

2. Over medium heat, quick fry the bacon until crispy then reserve on a plate. Set the pan on fire again to fry garlic and shallots for 30 seconds

3. Stir in apple cider vinegar, Brussels sprouts, and seasoning to cook for five minutes. Add the bacon to cook for five minutes then stir in the butter and set a hole at the center

4. Crash the eggs to the pan and let cook fully. Enjoy

Gluten-Free Pancakes

Prep Time: 5 min

Cook Time: 2 min

Serve: 2

Ingredients:

- 6 eggs

- 1 cup low-fat cream cheese

- 1 1/12; teaspoons baking powder

- 1 scoop protein powder

- 1/4 cup almond meal

- 1/4 teaspoon salt

Directions:

1. Combine dry ingredients in a food processor. Add the eggs one after another and then the cream cheese. Mix it well.

2. Lightly grease a skillet with cooking spray and place over medium- high heat. Pour the batter into the pan. Turn the pan gently to create round pancakes.

3. Cook for about 2 minutes on each side. Serve pancakes with your favorite topping.

Mushroom & Spinach Omelet

Prep Time: 20 min

Cook Time: 20 min

Serve: 3

Ingredients:

- 2 tablespoons butter, divided

- 6-8 fresh mushrooms, sliced

- 5 ounces Chives, chopped, optional

- Salt and pepper, to taste

- 1 handful baby spinach, about 1/2 ounce

- Pinch garlic powder

- 4 eggs, beaten

- 1-ounce shredded Swiss cheese

Directions:

1. In a very large saucepan, sauté the mushrooms in one tablespoon of butter until soft. Season with salt, pepper, and garlic. Remove the mushrooms from the pan and keep warm. Heat the remaining tablespoon of butter in the same skillet over medium heat.

1. Beat the eggs with a little salt and pepper and add to the hot butter. Turn the pan over to coat the entire bottom of the pan with egg. Once the egg is almost out, place the cheese over the middle of the tortilla.

2. Fill the cheese with spinach leaves and hot mushrooms. Let cook for about a minute for the spinach to start to wilt. Fold the tortilla's empty side carefully over the filling and slide it onto a plate and sprinkle with chives, if desired.

3. Alternatively, you can make two tortillas using half the mushroom, spinach, and cheese filling in each.

Avocado Spread

Prep Time: 5 min

Cook Time: 0 min

Serve: 8

Ingredients:

- 2 avocados, peeled, pitted and roughly chopped

- 1 tbsp. sun-dried tomatoes, chopped

- 2 tbsp. lemon juice

- 3 tbsp. cherry tomatoes, chopped

- ¼ cup red onion, chopped

- 1 tsp. oregano, dried

- 2 tbsp. parsley, chopped

- 4 kalamata olives, pitted and chopped

- A pinch of salt and black pepper

Directions:

1. Put the avocados in a bowl and mash with a fork.

2. Add the rest of the ingredients, stir to combine and serve as a morning spread.

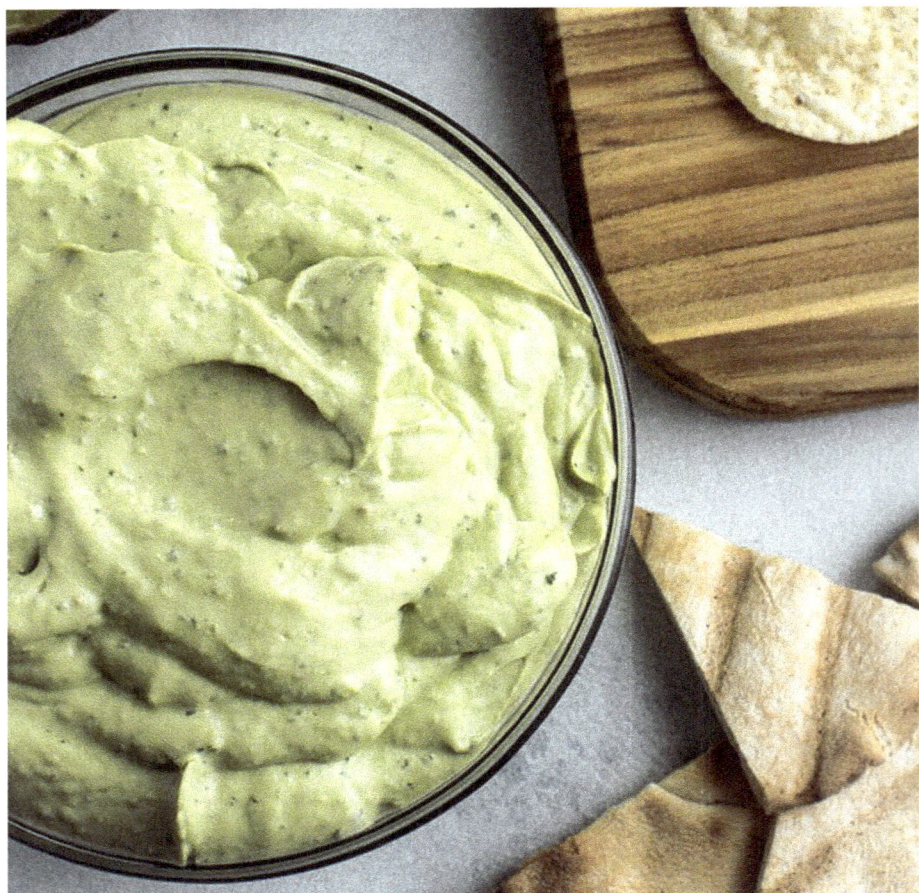

Artichokes and Cheese Omelet

Prep Time: 10 min

Cook Time: 8 min

Serve: 1

Ingredients:

- 1 tsp. avocado oil

- 1 tbsp. almond milk

- 2 eggs, whisked

- A pinch of salt and black pepper

- 2 tbsp. tomato, cubed

- 2 tbsp. kalamata olives, pitted and sliced

- 1 artichoke heart, chopped

- 1 tbsp. tomato sauce

- 1 tbsp. feta cheese, crumbled

Directions:

1. In a bowl, combine the eggs with the milk, salt, pepper and the rest of the ingredients except the avocado oil and whisk well.

2. Heat a pan with the avocado oil over medium-high heat, add the omelet mix, spread into the pan, cook for 4 minutes, flip, cook for 4 minutes more, transfer to a plate and serve.

Walnut Poached Eggs

Prep Time: 10 min

Cook Time: 10 min

Serve: 2

Ingredients:

- 2 slices whole grain bread toasted

- 1 oz sun-dried tomato, sliced

- 1 tbsp. cream cheese

- 1/3 tsp. minced garlic

- 2 slices prosciutto

- 2 eggs

- 1 tbsp. walnuts

- ½ cup fresh basil

- 1 oz Parmesan, grated

- 3 tbsp. olive oil

- ¼ tsp. ground black pepper

- 1 cup water, for cooking

Directions:

1. Pour water in the saucepan and bring it to boil. Then crack eggs in the boiling water and cook them for 3-4 minutes or until the egg whites are white. Meanwhile, churn together minced garlic and cream cheese.

2. Spread the bread slices with the cream cheese mixture. Top them with the sun-dried tomatoes. Make the pesto sauce: Blend together ground black pepper, Parmesan, olive oil, and basil. When the mixture is homogenous, pesto is cooked.

3. Carefully transfer the poached eggs over the sun-dried tomatoes and sprinkle with pesto sauce. The poached eggs should be hot while serving.

Almond Cream Cheese Bake

Prep Time: 10 min

Cook Time: 2 h

Serve: 4

Ingredients:

- 1 cup cream cheese
- 4 tbsp. honey
- 1 oz almonds, chopped
- ½ tsp. vanilla extract
- 3 eggs, beaten
- 1 tbsp. semolina

Directions:

1. Put beaten eggs in the mixing bowl. Add cream cheese, semolina, and vanilla extract. Blend the mixture with the help of the hand mixer until it is fluffy.

2. After this, add chopped almonds and mix up the mass well. Transfer the cream cheese mash in the non-sticky baking mold. Flatten the surface of the cream cheese mash well. Preheat the oven to 325°F. Cook the breakfast for 2 hours.

3. The meal is cooked when the surface of the mash is light brown. Chill the cream cheese mash little and sprinkle with honey.

Chili Egg Cups

Prep Time: 15 min

Cook Time: 15 min

Servings: 4

Ingredients:

- 1 tsp. chives, chopped

- 4 eggs

- 1 tsp. tomato paste

- 1 tbsp. Plain yogurt

- ½ tsp. butter, softened

- ¼ tsp. chili flakes

- ½ oz Cheddar cheese, shredded

Directions:

1. Preheat the oven to 365°F. Brush the muffin molds with the softened butter from inside.

2. Then mix up together Plain yogurt with chili flakes and tomato paste. Crack the eggs in the muffin molds.

3. After this, carefully place the tomato paste mixture over the eggs and top with Cheddar cheese. Sprinkle the eggs with chili flakes and place in the preheated oven.

4. Cook the egg cups for 15 minutes. Then check if the eggs are solid and remove them from the oven.

5. Chill the egg cups till the room temperature and gently remove from the muffin molds.

Dill Eggs Mix

Prep Time: 10 min

Cook Time: 15 min

Serve: 2

Ingredients:

- 2 eggs

- 2 oz Feta cheese

- 1 tsp. fresh dill, chopped

- 1 tsp. butter

- ½ tsp. olive oil

- ¼ tsp. onion powder

- ¼ tsp. chili flakes

Directions:

1. Toss butter in the skillet. Add olive oil and bring to boil.

2. After this, crack the eggs in the skillet. Sprinkle them with chili flakes and onion powder. Then preheat the oven to 360°F.

3. Transfer the skillet with eggs in the oven and cook for 10 minutes. Then crumble Feta cheese and sprinkle it over the eggs. Bake the eggs for 5 minutes more.

Hummus and Tomato Sandwich

Prep Time: 10 min

Cooking Time: 2 min

Serve: 3

Ingredients:

- 6 whole grain bread slices
- 1 tomato
- 3 Cheddar cheese slices
- ½ tsp. dried oregano
- 1 tsp. green chili paste
- ½ red onion, sliced
- 1 tsp. lemon juice
- 1 tbsp. hummus
- 3 lettuce leaves

Directions:

1. Slice tomato into 6 slices. In the shallow bowl mix up together dried oregano, green chili paste, lemon juice, and hummus.

2. Spread 3 bread slices with the chili paste mixture. After this, place the sliced tomatoes on them. Add sliced onion, Cheddar cheese, and lettuce leaves.

3. Cover the lettuce leaves with the remaining bread slices to get the sandwiches. Preheat the grill to 365°F. Grill the sandwiches for 2 minutes.

Buttery Pancakes

Prep Time: 10 min

Cook Time: 10 min

Servings: 5

Ingredients:

- 1 cup wheat flour, whole-grain
- 1 tsp. baking powder
- 1 tsp. lemon juice
- 3 eggs, beaten
- ¼ cup Splenda
- 1 tsp. vanilla extract
- 1/3 cup blueberries
- 1 tbsp. olive oil
- 1 tsp. butter
- 1/3 cup milk

Directions:

1. In the mixer bowl, combine baking powder, wheat flour, lemon juice, eggs, Splenda, vanilla extract, milk, and olive oil. Blend the liquid until it is smooth and homogenous.

2. After this, toss the butter in the skillet and melt it. With the spoon's help pour the pancake batter in the hot skillet and flatten it in the shape of the pancake.

3. Sprinkle the pancake with the blueberries gently and cook for 1.5 minutes over the medium heat. Then flip the pancake onto another side and cook it for 30 seconds more.

4. Repeat the same steps with all remaining batter and blueberries. Transfer the cooked pancakes in the serving plate.

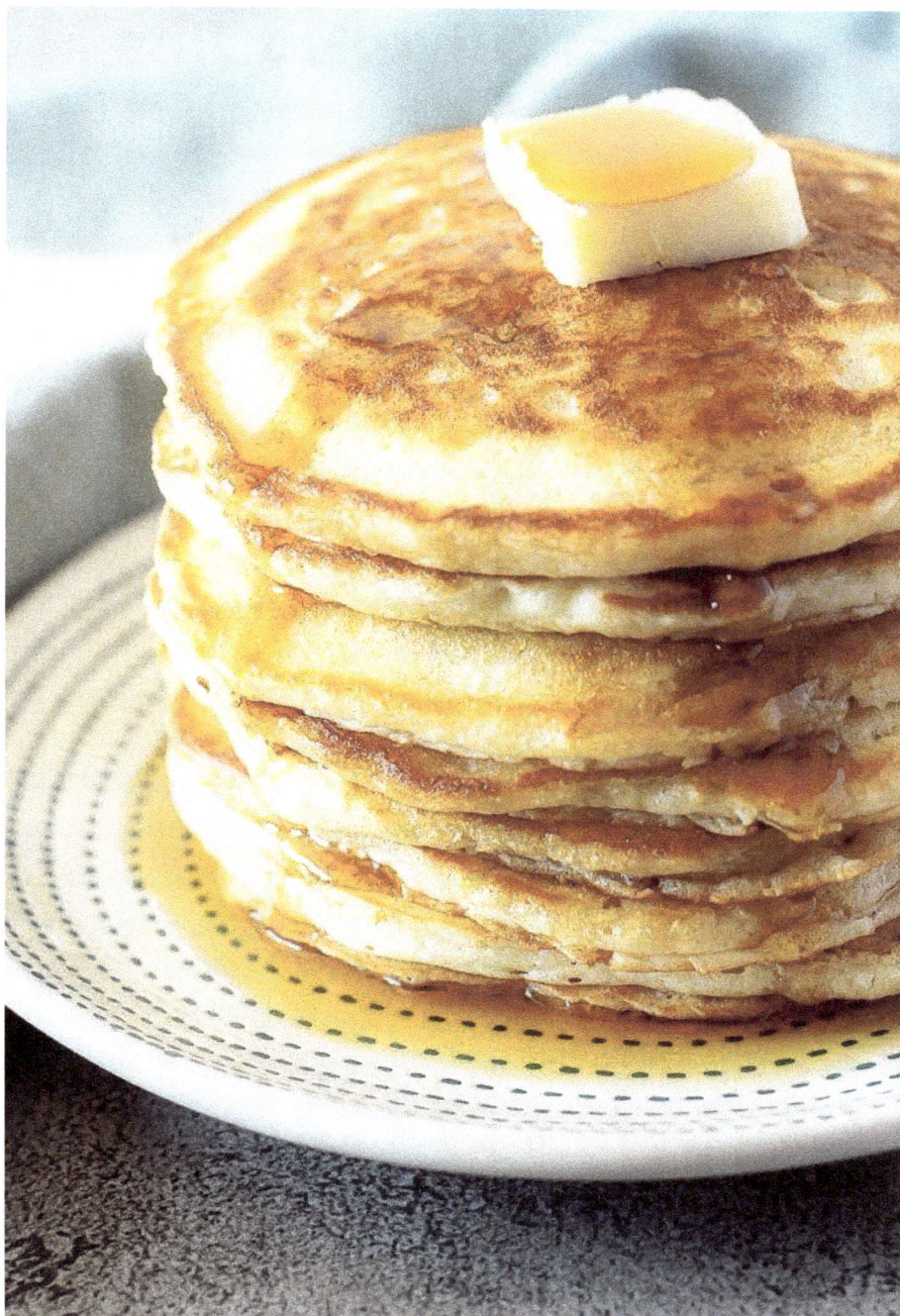

Cream Olive Muffins

Prep Time: 15 min

Cook Time: 20 min

Serve: 6

Ingredients:

- ½ cup quinoa, cooked
- 2 oz Feta cheese, crumbled
- 2 eggs, beaten
- 3 kalamata olives, chopped
- ¾ cup heavy cream
- 1 tomato, chopped
- 1 tsp. butter, softened
- 1 tbsp. wheat flour, whole grain
- ½ tsp. salt

Directions:

1. In the mixing bowl whisk eggs and add Feta cheese. Then add chopped tomato and heavy cream.

2. After this, add wheat flour, salt, and quinoa. Then add kalamata olives and mix up the ingredients with the help of the spoon. Brush the muffin molds with the butter from inside.

3. Transfer quinoa mixture in the muffin molds and flatten it with the spatula or spoon's help if needed.

4. Cook the muffins in the preheated to 355°F oven for 20 minutes.

Herbed Fried Eggs

Prep Time: 6 min

Cook Time: 7 min

Serve: 2

Ingredients:

- 4 eggs

- 1 tbsp. butter

- ½ tsp. chives, chopped

- ½ tsp. fresh parsley, chopped

- 1/3 tsp. fresh dill, chopped

- ¾ tsp. sea salt

Directions:

1. Toss butter in the skillet and bring it to boil. Then crack the eggs in the coiled butter and sprinkle with sea salt.

2. Cook the eggs with the closed lid for 2 minutes over the medium heat. Then open the lid and sprinkle them with parsley, dill, and chives.

3. Cook the eggs for 3 minutes more over the medium heat. 4. Carefully transfer the cooked meal in the plate. Use the wooden spatula for this step.

Chili Scramble

Prep Time: 15 min

Cook Time: 15 min

Serve: 4

Ingredients:

- 3 tomatoes

- 4 eggs

- ¼ tsp. of sea salt

- ½ chili pepper, chopped

- 1 tbsp. butter

- 1 cup water, for cooking

Directions:

1. Pour water in the saucepan and bring it to boil. Then remove water from the heat and add tomatoes. Let the tomatoes stay in the hot water for 2-3 minutes.

2. After this, remove the tomatoes from water and peel them. Place butter in theee pan and melt it.

3. Add chopped chili pepper and fry it for 3 minutes over the medium heat. Then chop the peeled tomatoes and add into the chili peppers.

4. Cook the vegetables for 5 minutes over the medium heat. Stir them from time to time. After this, add sea salt and crack the eggs Stir (scramble) the eggs well with the fork's help and cook them for 3 minutes over the medium heat.

Couscous and Chickpeas Bowls

Prep Time: 10 min

Cook Time: 6 min

Serve: 4

Ingredients:

- ¾ cup whole wheat couscous
- 1 yellow onion, chopped
- 1 tbsp. olive oil
- 1 cup water
- 2 garlic cloves, minced
- 15 oz. canned chickpeas, drained and rinsed
- A pinch of salt and black pepper
- 15 oz. canned tomatoes, chopped
- 14 oz. canned artichokes, drained and chopped
- ½ cup Greek olives, pitted and chopped
- ½ tsp. oregano, dried

- 1 tbsp. lemon juice

Directions:

1. Put the water in a pot, bring to a boil over medium heat, add the couscous, stir, take off the heat, cover the pan, leave aside for 10 minutes and fluff with a fork.

2. Heat a pan with the oil over medium-high heat, add the onion and sauté for 2 minutes. Add the rest of the ingredients, toss and cook for 4 minutes more.

3. Add the couscous, toss, divide into bowls and serve for breakfast.

Anti-Inflammatory

Blueberry Smoothie

Prep Time: 5 min

Cook Time: 5 min

Serve: 1

Ingredients:

- Almond milk (1 cup)

- Frozen banana (1)

- Frozen blueberries (2/3-1 cup)

- Leafy greens/spinach (2 handfuls)

- Almond butter (1 tbsp.)

- Cinnamon (.25 tsp.)

- Cayenne pepper (.125-.25 tsp.)

- Optional: Maca powder (1 tsp.)

Directions:

1. Combine each of the fixings using a high-powered blender. Mix thoroughly until creamy and serve in a chilled glass.

Cherry - Pomegranate Smoothie Bow - Gluten-Free & Vegetarian

Prep Time: 5 min

Cook Time: 5 min

Serve: 4

Ingredients:

- Frozen dark sweet cherries (16 oz. bag)

- 2% Plain Greek yogurt (1.5 cups)

- Pomegranate juice (.75 cup)

- 2% milk (.33 cup (+) more as needed)

- Ground cinnamon (.75 tsp.)

- Vanilla extract (1 tsp.)

- Fresh pomegranate seeds (.5 cup)

- Chopped pistachios (.5 cup)

- Ice cubes (6)

Directions:

1. Chop the pistachios or purchase (arils) found in the produce section of the market. If you are using the whole fruit, remove the seeds underwater in a container to float to the top.

2. Add the fixings into a blender (ice, milk, cinnamon, vanilla, juice, yogurt, and cherries). Pulse until it's creamy smooth. Use a little extra milk to thin the texture to get it to the desired consistency.

3. Pour the prepared smoothie into for dishes and top with two tbsp. of the chopped pistachios and two tbsp. of the seeds. Serve it immediately.

Breakfast Banana Green Smoothie

Prep Time: 5 min

Cook Time: 5 min

Serve: 1

Ingredients:

- 2 cups baby spinach leaves or 1 banana

- ¾ cup plain Fat-free Greek yogurt, or to taste

- ¾ cup ice

- 2 tbsp. honey

- 1 carrot

Directions:

1. Put spinach, banana, carrot, yogurt, ice, and honey in a blender; blend until smooth. Enjoy!

Strawberry Oatmeal

Breakfast Smoothie

Prep Time: 5 min

Cook Time: 5 min

Serve: 2

Ingredients:

- 1 cup soy milk

- ½ cup rolled oats

- 1 banana, broken into chunks

- 14 frozen strawberries

- ½ tsp. vanilla extract

- 1 ½ tsp. white sugar

Directions:

1. In a blender, combine soy milk, oats, banana and strawberries. Add vanilla and sugar if desired. Blend until smooth. Pour into glasses and serve.

Kale and Banana

Smoothie

Prep Time: 5 min

Cook Time: 5 min

Serve: 1

Ingredients:

- 1 banana

- 2 cups chopped kale

- ½ cup light unsweetened soy milk

- 1 tbsp. flax seeds

- 1 tsp. maple syrup

Directions:

1. Place the banana, kale, soy milk, flax seeds, and maple syrup into a blender. Cover, and puree until smooth. Serve over ice.

Pumpkin Pie Fall Smoothie

Prep Time: 5 min

Cook Time: 0 min

Serve: 3

Ingredients:

- 1 cup almond milk

- 1 tsp. agave syrup

- 1 cup pumpkin puree

- 2 tsp. cinnamon

- 1 apple, cored Dried cranberries

Directions:

1. Combine all ingredients except cranberries in blender and blend until smooth. Top with cranberries and enjoy.

Green Tart Smoothie

Prep Time: 5 min

Cook Time: 5 min

Serve: 1

Ingredients:

- 2 cups fresh kale
- 1 cup water
- 2 large stalks of celery, chopped
- ½ cucumber, chopped
- 1/3 grapefruit
- 1 cup frozen pineapple

Directions:

1. Blend kale and water until smooth. Add remaining ingredients, and blend until smooth. Enjoy!

Gluten-Free Pancakes

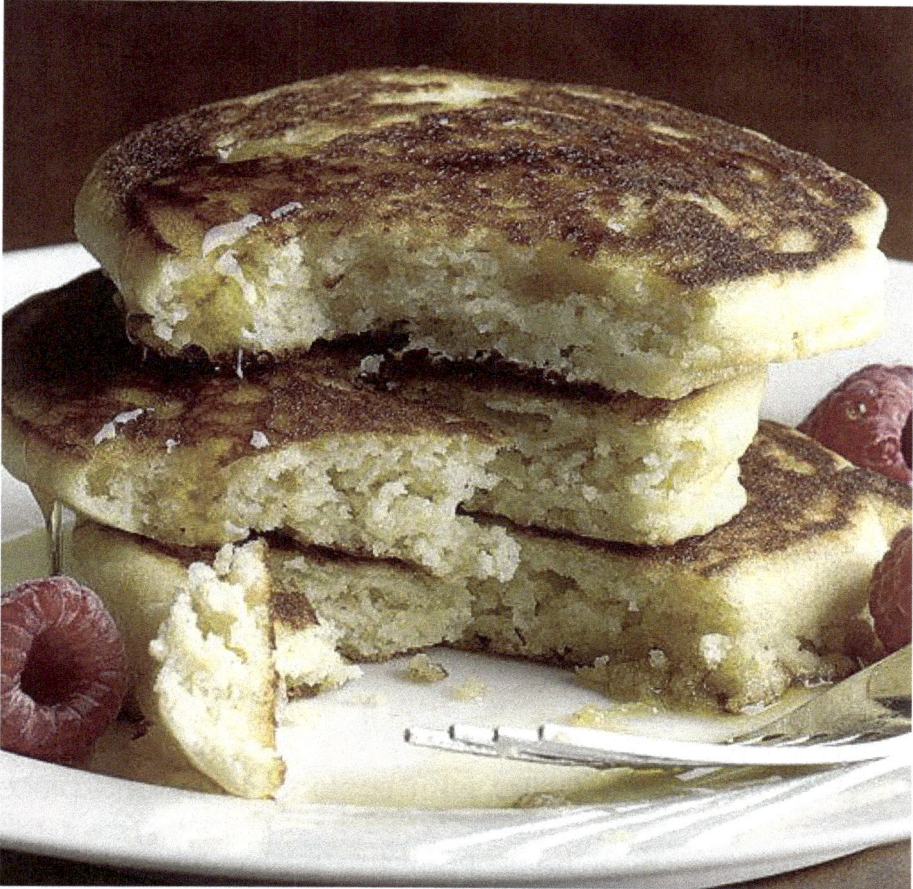

Prep Time: 5 min

Cook Time: 2 min

Serve: 2

Ingredients:

- 6 eggs

- 1 cup low-fat cream cheese

- 1 1/12; teaspoons baking powder

- 1 scoop protein powder

- 1/4 cup almond meal

- ¼ teaspoon salt

-

Directions:

1. Combine dry ingredients in a food processor. Add the eggs one after another and then the cream cheese. Mix it well.

2. Lightly grease a skillet with cooking spray and place over medium- high heat. Pour the batter into the pan. Turn the pan gently to create round pancakes.

3. Cook for about 2 minutes on each side. Serve pancakes with your favorite topping.

Summer Stone Fruit Smoothie

Prep Time: 5 min

Cook Time: 0 min

Serve: 2

Ingredients:

- ½ cup Greek yogurt

- 1 plum, pit removed, flesh roughly chopped

- 1 peach

- 1 nectarine, pit removed, flesh roughly chopped

- ½ cup blueberries, fresh or frozen

Directions:

1. Combine all ingredients in blender and blend until smooth. Enjoy!

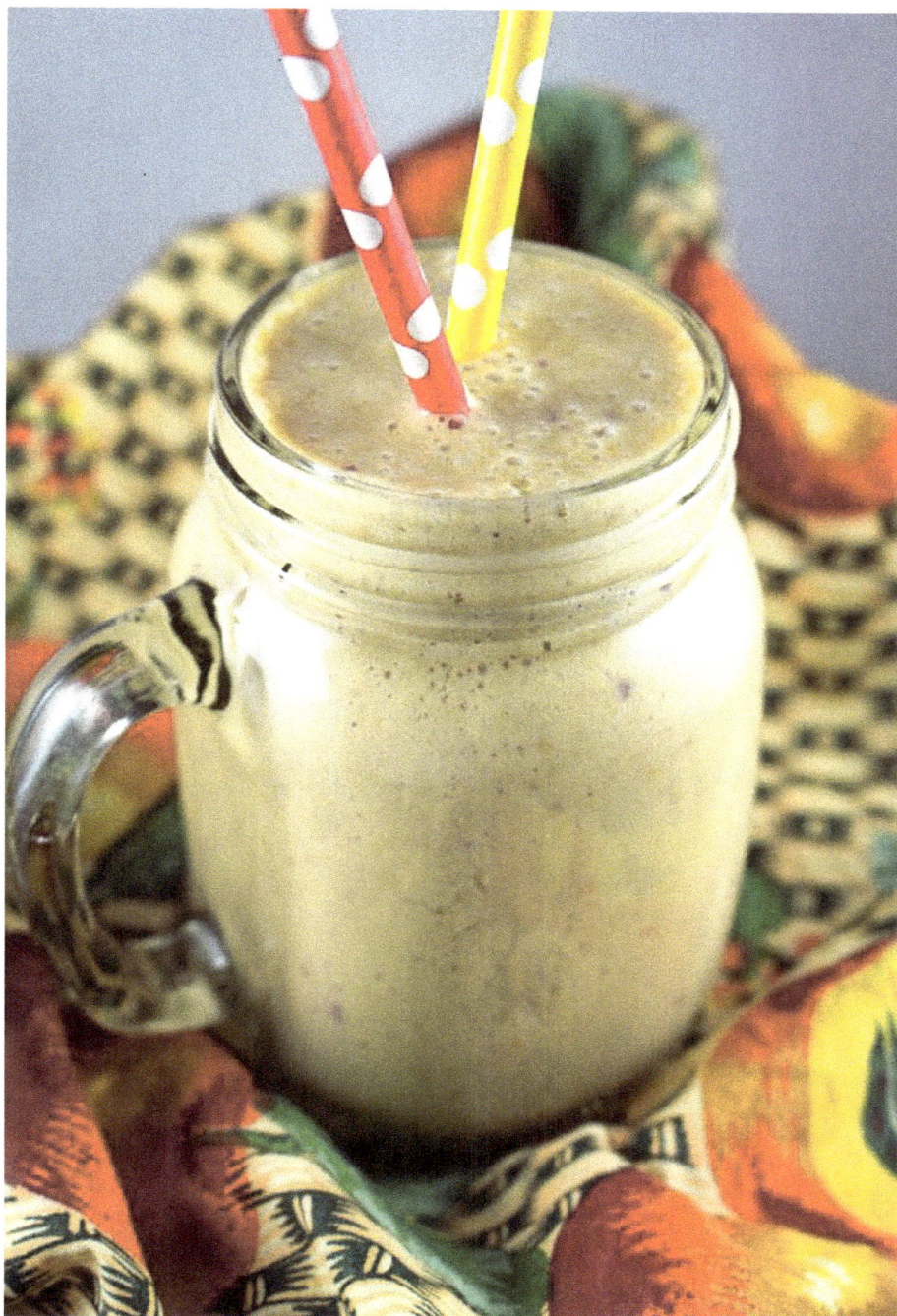

www.ingramcontent.com/pod-product-compliance
Lightning Source LLC
Chambersburg PA
CBHW071108030426

42336CB00013BA/1994